SHATTERED DREAMS
— AND —
BROKEN HEARTS

SHATTERED DREAMS
— AND —
BROKEN HEARTS

Depression, Suicide, Death,
and the Pain It Leaves Behind

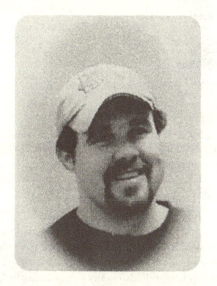

LINDA J. STILSON

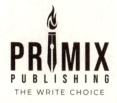

Primix Publishing
11620 Wilshire Blvd
Suite 900, West Wilshire Center, Los Angeles, CA, 90025
www.primixpublishing.com
Phone: 1-800-538-5788

© 2023 Linda J. Stilson. All rights reserved.
No part of this book may be reproduced, stored in a retrieval system, or transmitted by any means without the written permission of the author.

Published by Primix Publishing: 07/14/2023

ISBN: 978-1-957676-62-3(sc)
ISBN: 978-1-957676-63-0(hc)
ISBN: 978-1-957676-64-7(e)

Library of Congress Control Number: 2023911784

Any people depicted in stock imagery provided by iStock are models, and such images are being used for illustrative purposes only.

Certain stock imagery © iStock.

Because of the dynamic nature of the Internet, any web addresses or links contained in this book may have changed since publication and may no longer be valid. The views expressed in this work are solely those of the author and do not necessarily reflect the views of the publisher, and the publisher hereby disclaims any responsibility for them.

Photo on front cover was taken at the Grand Canyon by Linda of her son standing on the edge.

Dedication

I dedicate this book in loving memory of my precious son, Michael Joseph Stilson, who committed suicide on December 20, 2004. I dedicate this book to all of the children that have died by suicide. No one can truly know the amount of pain that one can handle or why they felt they had no other way to continue to live. May they be at peace with the Lord. May we learn more about the signs and treatment of suicide and hopefully prevent others that feel their life isn't worth living.

I also dedicate this book to my grandchildren that have been very supportive and caring of me during my loss. Thank you to the twins who were able to go with me on my healing trip to NC and to be with me when we scattered my son's ashes with my son's wife and family in New York.

I also wish to dedicate this book to the parents on the online support group, POS (Parents of Suicide) for all their love and support that they have given me during this tragic loss. Only those that have gone through the loss of a child by suicide can truly understand the pain and tragic loss that we feel on this horrible journey we are on.

I thank all my friends and neighbors that have been there for me during my losses and helping to see that I don't fall apart. I always felt the Lord brought me here to Arizona for a reason, and I think it was because he knew what my future was going to hold and that I would need a lot of friends and neighbors to keep me busy.

Thank you to my family for their love and support.

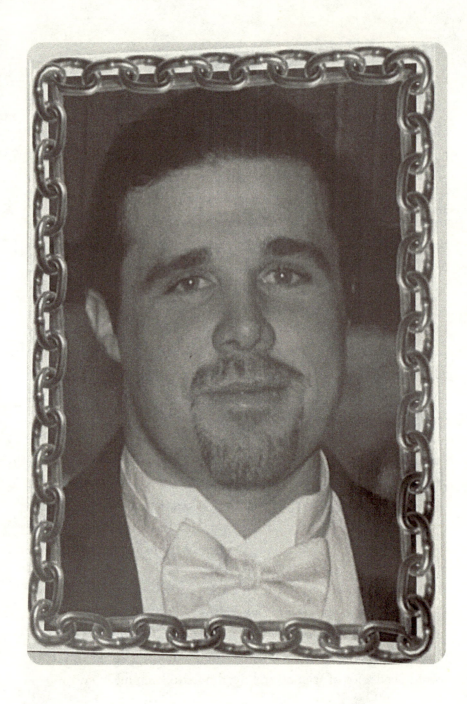

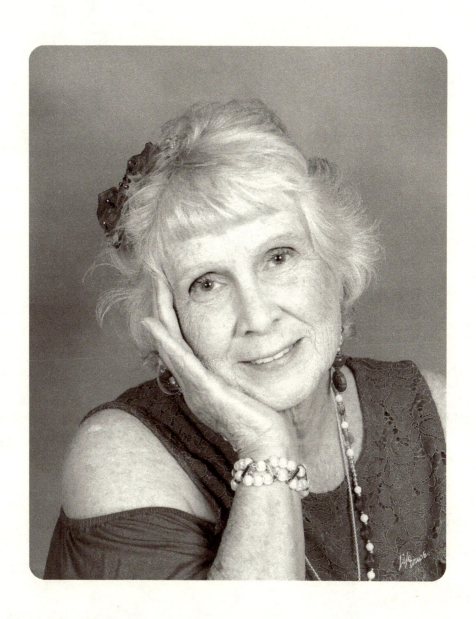

Introduction

On Saturday, February 6, 1971 at 3:15am I gave birth to a 10 pound 13 ounce, 22 1/211 baby boy. I named him Michael Joseph because it meant "like unto God.an addition". He was my only birth child and meant the world to me. On December 20, 2004 I was notified by police that my son had committed suicide.

I had just lost my husband, Bill, on Feb. 2, 2001 from cancer after 26 years of marriage. I never thought that I would ever be where I am now grieving because my only birth child committed suicide. I still find it hard to accept that my son is really dead, let alone say the word. One never is prepared for that, nor do they feel it will ever happen to them. Our children are to bury us, not the other way around. The problem is that for many of us, we either didn't see or know the signs, or our child kept it hidden from us. That needs to be changed. We need to learn more about suicide, as well as the medical conditions that lead up to suicide. We must change the way people think about suicide being a sin. Only God can judge us and I know that my God is a loving and forgiving God and that he held out more love and compassion for the sick, the poor, and the troubled.

Although my son was diagnosed with ADDH when he was in first grade, I think his problem was more of being bipolar as I now realize the signs as similar to what he had growing up. He was moody and lacked coping skills. He was a risk taker as well as impulsive to the extent he didn't think about consequences. When he was frustrated he talked of dying and always said he wouldn't live to be 25, then 35. Why didn't I know those were signs of a serious illness? I took him to the doctors often enough. Why didn't they? Why did they automatically diagnose him with ADDH? Michael had a high

IQ and was bored with school because he wasn't challenged enough, even though he had a reading disability, and was dyslexic. He had a poor self- esteem and got discouraged very easily.

Michael was a very loving, caring young man who had a gift for bringing a smile to your face when he entered the room. He loved children and always made them feel important. Michael graduated from high school and went into the construction job field and was well liked by many. He moved to Raleigh and worked there for a few years and then moved back to NY to be closer to his girlfriend. They were married May 17, 2002 and bought a house in October. They came out to visit me in Arizona, April 2004. In July 2004 my son called to say goodbye. He was going to commit suicide. There were too many things going on in his life that were overwhelming to him. He had lost a job, started another one which laid him off in two weeks, fell off a roof 28 feet, no medical insurance, finances only mounting, raising teenage stepchildren. As much as he loved his wife and his stepchildren and worried about their well-being, he just wasn't able to handle the pressures. He prided his financial stability, so when things started going wrong he sank into depression and started drinking more to dull his inner pain and became an angry person.

He was not a forgiving person when he was rejected or hurt, and he felt rejected by many people over the past years that he had admired and respected and he took it personally. He couldn't get past the hurt. He was such a proud and stubborn young man. Due to his depression I wasn't able to get him to think past it or make the first move to mend those relationships. Unfortunately there were just too many issues at once and he lacked the coping skills to be capable of dealing with them. I helped him out with finances and was told that things were going much better. I was going to move back East to be closer to him. I will never know if that was true or if that was what he wanted me to think. He knew how much it hurt me when he had threatened suicide. I thought that was the worst thing to happen until the day the police came to say he had committed suicide.

In December he told me he was having a special gift made for me for Christmas to express how much he loved me and to thank me for always loving him and being there for him. His gift arrived as the police were leaving from telling me the news of his death. So much is unknown about that night and what led up to it. I can only say that he isn't here to defend himself or explain why and blaming anyone isn't going to bring him back. On the night that Michael died, he drank an excessive amount of hard liquor at a Christmas party. His autopsy report showed that his blood alcohol count was 2.6 and showed no drugs of any kind in his body. I never approved of his drinking as his father and I didn't drink or smoke and lived a Christian life. I had pleaded with him to stop his drinking because it only made his depression worse and didn't solve his problems.

I feel sorry for the pain my son's death caused his wife and his stepchildren, as no one deserved to have to witness his death. Unfortunately he was more troubled than he let on or we knew, and he felt he couldn't face the future. Perhaps if his wife and I had known more about depression and Bipolar Disorder, we might have been able to get Michael to accept treatment and he would be here now. I had urged him to see a doctor and that I would pay for it, but he wouldn't accept any more help. Being an adult, it was still his choice to accept help and to continue with the treatment. Depression and Bipolar Disorder are both illnesses and although they may not be cured, they are treatable, but if left untreated.most often leads to suicide.

One moment of happiness spent together to lives torn apart, in just a matter of minutes from a moment of anger; where love once triumphed. His death left pain and heartache to those he left behind: For a mother, there is no greater loss. A mother loves from the time a child is growing inside her until she dies. For his wife and his stepchildren whose lives have been torn apart. For his friends and family, who are left without his wit, humor and friendship. Little did he know how much he was loved, because in his depression he felt alone.

I have expressed my feelings of my grief in poetry and I hope that they bring comfort and understanding to others that have suffered such a loss, or those that may be thinking of suicide. Our children are the future of the world and we need to help them. Check out the recommended websites and become familiar with the signs and what to look for as you never know when you may need them.

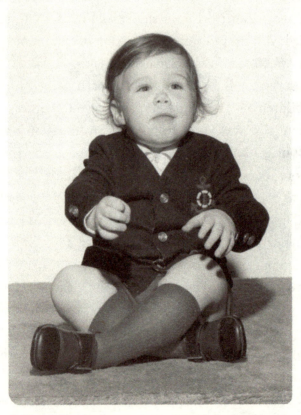

Mike at 18 months wearing suit made by his favorite
Aunt Dorothy Burdick wearing the red boots that were my
Brother Fran's when he was young.

My Prayer

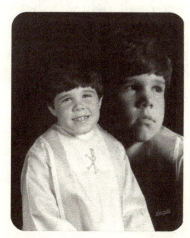

Michael's 1st Communion at 8 yrs old

I pray for peace for my son who died.
I pray for peace for those who cried.
I pray for healing from the pain we're in.
I pray for those who treat suicide as a sin.
I pray for forgiveness for the signs no one saw.
I pray for the ones who never bothered to call.
I pray for forgiveness for guilt one may feel.
I pray for understanding that hearts will soon heal.
I pray for awareness of depression that I now know.
I pray for healing for depression for those who are feeling low.
I pray that their friends will be there with love to show.
I pray for peace for those whose troubles take their tow.
I pray for peace for those on POS for all you do.
My peace to you and God Bless You.

If tears could build a stairway
and memories were a lane,

I would walk right up to heaven
to bring you home again

No farewell words were spoken
No time to say goodbye

You were gone before I knew it,
and only GOD knows why.

My heart still aches in sadness,
and secret tears still flow.

What it means to lose you,
no one will ever know.

Author Unknown

Suicide is not chosen. It happens when pain exceeds the resources to cope with the pain.

My Precious Michael, How Tragic Your Death Was For Me

My dearest Michael, how tragic your death was for me.
Forgive me for missing your signs, why didn't I see.
I feel so sad that you felt so helpless and blue.
Your pain overwhelming that it only consumed you.
How alone you must have felt on that tragic day.
Left feeling so hopeless, with nothing to say.
I do wish you had called or reached out to me.
I could have hugged you so dearly, my Michael, you see.
I miss you so badly, my heart it does ache.
So deeply it feels like it surely will break.
My dreams for your future have drifted away.
It seems so unreal that it feels like a nightmare or play.
Yet I've prayed you would walk through that door some day.
As I'd hug you so tightly; I have so much to say.
My handsome, young Michael; so precious to me.
Your death left me broken from what life near you was going to be.
How sadly I feel now that you are no longer here.
I won't get to see you until I die and I'm there.
With you and the Lord, may you now be at peace.
May his love now surround you, your loneliness cease.
How I prayed that you would reach out to our Lord above,
Like Footprints in the Sand he was there for you with love.
He died for your sins so you would be free.
You just needed to call out to loved ones that he gave to thee.
So now I must treasure my memories of my life once with you.

Before your life became so mixed up and left you broken in two.
My precious Michael, I miss your smile and your laughter,
And will always love and miss you.

How deep your loss has left me, a mother without her child.
Love U4ever, Mom

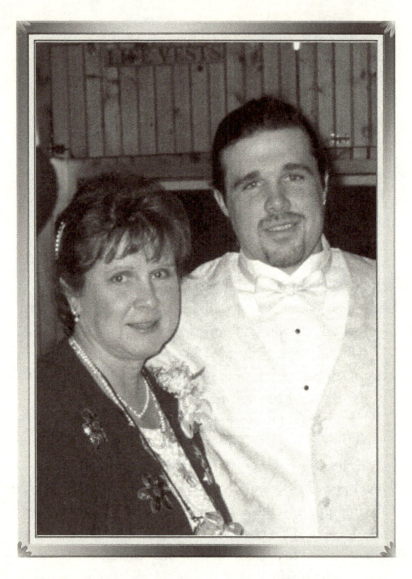

Why Did You Have to Drink Your Life Away?

Why did you have to drink your life away?
Why couldn't you have found a way to stay?
What was it made you think your life was bad?
What turned you inside out and made you feel so sad?

Why couldn't you see how many friends you had?
Why didn't you turn to one of them when you were sad?
What made you feel they wouldn't care you were hurting inside?
What good did it do to hide your feelings
and the pain inside to hide?

You left behind a family, stepchildren and a wife, Why did
they have to see your anguish and watch you take your life?
Now their life is traumatized by the
tragedy and of the terrible sight,
The haunting memories of the gunshot
on that tragic, December night.

The pain of your death and leaving us will never go away.
No matter how much we cry, or how often that we will pray.
Not having you here with us has left our hearts broken in two.
Why couldn't you see how unhappy we'd
be, leaving us without you?

I wish I had known that you thought about suicide.
Or known what to look for.the signs that you'd hide.
That what you told me was what you wanted me to hear,
Because hurting me was more than you could ever bear.

I ask God to help us to heal our pain,
To not let our heartache leave us feeling insane.
To help us accept that we were unable to help you,
Those choices you made were decided by you.

That alcohol changed you and altered your mind.
Magnifying loneliness and sadness; leaving your life here behind.
If only you had reached out, for a friend to hold your hand,
And remembered God was with you,
like the footprints in the sand.

Please know that I forgive you, for leaving us behind,
I'm sorry that you felt that life on earth was treating you unkind.
I pray that you embrace the Lord and feel his love for you.
Cause he was always there for you, that's why he died for you.

When did you change from that sweet child of mine?

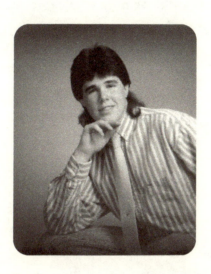

Your eyes how they sparkled
And how they did shine
Your laughter and humor
Touched more hearts than mine
Your antics and mischief
How they kept me running
Your lies of denial
How sly and so cunning
A sweet loving boy
With a heart of gold
Who should have lived longer
Until he was old
When did you change
From that sweet boy of mine?

How did we miss your depression
And not see the sign?
That suicide was the way
You saw to ending your pain
Now our hearts are broken
And our tears are like rain
The mystery of depression
And suicide unfolding
The unanswered questions
That seems so unending
My love could not shelter you
Or keep you from pain
So I pray that you find peace
With God in his reign
Let his love surround you
And fill your heart with glee
When I look in the sky for your star
Shining down on me.

Anger Has Its Hold on Me

Anger has its hold on me…
Ever since your life was taken you see.
I hate that you didn't walk away
From all the fighting that upset you that day.
I hate it that I wasn't there for you to turn to.
I hate the way your family mistreated you.
I hate it that you wasn't strong
To deal with all the things that went so wrong.
I hate that life for you was never an easy one.
I hate that you suffered for what other's had done.
I hate that my life is empty without you here.
I hate that God didn't take me to be with you there.
I hate that my family never made time to spend with you.
I hate that they hurt you and added to
your feelings of rejection too.
I hate that medical help was not financially available for you.
I hate that your pride prevented your accepting help too.
I hate that you felt death was the only way,
To ease your pain and you chose to die that day.
I hate that my Christmas now will be painful for me.
A constant reminder. that your life was taken tragically.
I hate that I have lost those most precious in my heart.
The pain of losing you has torn my world apart.
I hate that I've been hating, but I have never hated you.
I know that you were hurting and knew not what to do.
I hate that this anger has got a hold on me.
Another stage of grieving of what it's said to be.

I know I'll come to terms with it and work through all my pain.
I know holding onto anger, leaves nothing
whatsoever for me to gain.
Deep seated it will consume my life and tear my heart apart.
Unless I put it all to rest and work to mend my broken heart.
For I know it's wrong to let anger take a hold of me.
But sometimes in grief it isn't always easy for one to see.

The "Blaming Game" Is Where I'm At….

The "Blaming Game" is where I'm at.
What didn't I do, Did I do that?
What could I have done to keep you here?
Was it because I didn't live so near?
Didn't I raise you to know wrong from right?
That compromises are better than to argue and fight?
Did I neglect teaching you coping skills?
That sometimes it's necessary to take anti- depressant pills.
Why did you feel you had to become a man that's tough?
Why did you hide your emotions inside when times were rough?
Why didn't you reveal your sensitivity and have to be so proud?
Why didn't you listen when I told you crying for help was allowed?
I loved you no matter what you did, because I was proud of you.
It tore me apart to know that you were broken in two.
Why did you worry too much about how other's felt?
Your pain so deep inside, one couldn't see the welt.
Why didn't I speak out more with you to hear what I had to say?
Was it because I knew how mad you would
get and only turn me away?
Why couldn't I have searched for help for you?
I would have found it on the internet like I now do.
The answers were there on the websites, if I had only looked.
The constant searching for answers will only get you hooked.
Why didn't I just surf the web for help for you.
My ignorance only leaves me feeling like a fool.
Knowing it was as easy as www.suicide.com , you see.
I just hope that others won't make that mistake like me.

The stages of grief I'm going through now.
The gut-ripping pain of always wondering how!
They say it's all normal, emotions tearing us apart.
Time ticking slowly, as we wait to mend our broken heart.
A loving mother is what I had always wanted to be.
Now I am left without my child, with only my memory.
With one stage of grieving gone for me.
With another one to replace it, you see.

No Greater Loss

There is no greater… Loss on earth
Than the loss… You've given me.
No one can bring you…back to me.
You didn't share it…For us to see…

You kept it hidden.Inside from others
No one could see…not even me.
Life is a journey…We all must take
There are no promises…Except those we make

No one can walk your road…not even me.
When trouble arises…Creates a crisis
We all must learn to trust…The ones who love us
No one could make you see…not even me.

Chorus:
    There are people out there
    Who understand and care
    Reach out to those you love
    Say a prayer to God above
    Let them give you a helping hand
    Remember Footprints in the sand
    Tomorrow is another day
    Learn that death is not the way
    Get the help and do it today
    Suicide is not the way

Your death won't end the pain
Cause you only pass it on
To all the ones behind
They're the ones you left in pain.

No one's worth your dying
No amount of crying
No forgotten words one said
Isn't worth your being dead

Don't drown your sorrows
In drugs or booze
There will be a tomorrow
You have nothing to lose

Be strong and fight the urge
Call a friend and talk it out
Let the fears and pain emerge
Don't be afraid to cry it out

Chorus:

My Sister's Losses

There are no words one can express or say to someone who has lost four children, one was stillborn. My heart goes out to my sister, Pam Mayer Thompson. This is what she has to say:

My heart is broken and feels like I have a hole in it that will never heal. No parent should outlive their child, let alone four. The pain is unbearable. I know I have two remaining daughters, and I am thankful for them, but I will never forget the four that I have lost. I will always love and miss them. I pray my children are at peace with the Lord and pray that my faith will give me the strength to face each day and find purpose with life. I will treasure my memories and time I had with them.

Love always, Pam Mayer Thompson

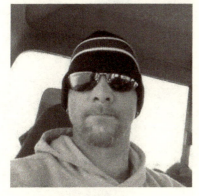

Richard Thompson
"Richie"

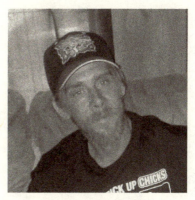

Frank Thompson
"Frankie"

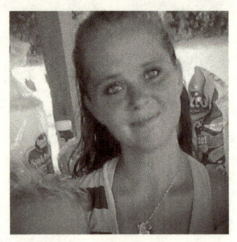

Kristen Thompson
Kristy

There is surely no greater loss than losing three of your five children. Prayers for healing for family and friends. Love Always, your sister, Linda.

I wish you were here so I wouldn't be missing you....

I miss my little boy making his birthday wish,
I miss my little boy, who loved to camp and fish,
I miss watching you play baseball and football,
I miss all the things we did together most of all.
I miss the camping trips and tubing we did,
I miss all the antics of my mischievous kid.
I miss all the fun things you did as a child,
I miss even the bad things you did when you were wild.
I miss the smile on your handsome face.
I miss your excitement after a winning NASCAR race.
I miss having you here for me to hug.
I miss the days we looked forward to.
I miss moving East to be closer to you.
I miss the dinners together watching you eat.
I miss your raiding my freezer for favorite treats.
I miss you waking in the morning to watch the sunrise.
I miss you opening your presents like a kid with shouts of surprise.
I miss hearing the tales of your antics and fun.
I miss having you near me...my dear precious son.
I miss you my son, and the love that you gave me.
I miss all the hugs and the way that things used to be.
I miss that the things that we planned will no longer be.
I miss you my son, without you is painful for me.
I wish you were here, so I wouldn't be missing you.

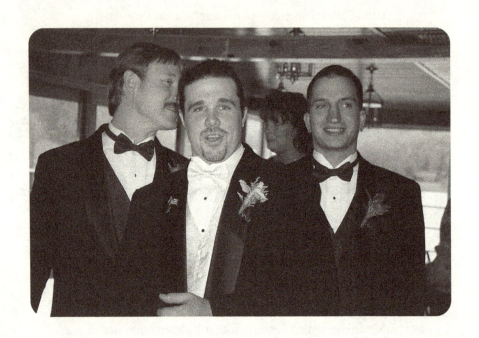

When Will My Sorrow Ever End?

When will my sorrow ever end?
When will my heartache start to mend?
When will the tears cease to fall?
When will I be able to see your pictures on the wall?

How do I accept that you are not here?
That when I go back East you won't be there?
How do I get by without your calls to me?
That plans we made together will never come to be.

I know not why your life was ended.
I know it was in your control for it to be mended.
I have accepted I did my best with you.
I gave you love and let you know it too.

So I must live my life one day by day,
Be strong and turn to God to pray.
That life for me will some day be,
Happy memories of you and your life with me!

The sorrow I feel losing you may never end.
The heartache will be here when it begins to mend.
The tears for you may lesson but still may fall.
The day will come when your pictures come off the wall.
When will my sorrow ever end?
The day that I stop loving you!

Mother's Day For Me In Eternity

I don't know why you had to die.
Didn't you know it would make me cry?
Leaving me here to mourn my loss.
Not knowing why - What was the cause?

What was the reason that you were so sad?
What made you feel your life was so bad?
Couldn't you have talked it out?
Told someone what it all was about?

I wish you knew it didn't have to be.
Things have a way of looking worse you see.
Sometimes there is no choice but walking away,
Wake up tomorrow to face another day.

Life is full of heartache and living with mistakes
One has to be strong and survive for other's sake.
Let those that love you help you work it out.
Pour out your feelings and give it a shout.

So here I am without my child to hug.
Deep in despair in this hole that I've dug.
Holding on to the hope tomorrow will be.
Mother's Day for me in eternity.

Mother's Day Without You I Cried
In memory of my son, Michael Joseph,
Who always remembered his mother on Mother's Day

Mother's Day was without my child this year.
The anticipation of this day was filled with dread and fear.
How was I to get through this day without you?
Knowing I wouldn't get your call made me blue.
Now I must find a different way,
To make special plans for my Mother's Day.
Just because you are not here...doesn't change a thing.
For all that Mother's Day represents or it brings.
I still carried you nine months and then gave birth.
To a big beautiful baby boy for all you were worth.
The joy of your birth was worth all the pain.
Which went away quicker than the weight I did gain.
So I will accept that I am always your mother.
That when you died, God didn't give you another.
You have only gone from here to Heaven to live on.
For I am still your mother; and you are still my son.
I can still remember you on Mother's Day.
I'll celebrate your memories in a special way.
The love you showed me all those years before you died.
Is the reason that on Mother's Day without you that I cried.

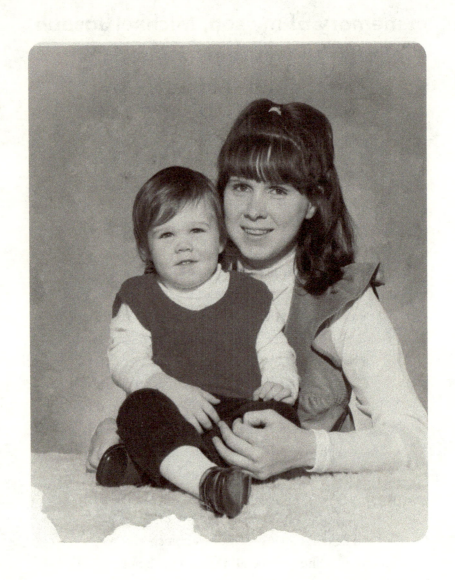

My Life Now Here Without You Today

I look for all the reasons
You're no longer here with me.
But none can bring me comfort
Knowing I will never see.
That handsome man, your eyes, your smile,
That you grew up to be.
The times we spent together
Or how thoughtful you were to me.
The marriage that I had hoped for you
Was not as it should be.
The problems grew too much for you,
The pain too much to see.
Hidden from those who loved you,
Made you feel so all alone.
If only you had reached out
Or called someone on the phone.
For now I'm in shock and denial,
That you are no longer here.
I guess it's because we lived apart
So far so I wasn't there.
It feels like you are on a trip somewhere,
And gone a month or two.
I guess it's easier for me
To think that way,
Than my life now here
Without you today.

Did I Do All that I Could?

Did I do all that I could?
To help you, my child, as any parent should.
This is the question that burdens me, Ever
since you died until eternity.
I need to accept that I gave all my love, That your life was not
in my control of. Your death was not my choice but yours.
That your pain is now gone and your spirit now soars.
Yet, though I know this, it still bothers me,
That I didn't know more or I didn't see.
How troubled your life was, too much for you to bear,
That you couldn't reach out to those who would care.
The mystery of depression still questions all, As more of our
loved ones stumble and fall. Awareness and prevention we must
attend to, So it doesn't end in suicide like it did with you.
We must educate ourselves more so we know all of the signs,
Learn about treatment for those troubled minds. Listen
with our hearts and learn to give out more hugs.
Depression isn't a sin to be hidden under a rug. So
I remind myself I gave unconditional love, To my
child who now lives with the Lord up above.
I did for my child as any good mother should.
I did do my best for my child of all that I could.

What Can I do To End My Grief?

What can I do to end my grief?
To end my pain and find relief.
I don't want to forget my love for you.
I just want to forget the pain and feeling blue.
When I wake in the morning light.
I want to enjoy the beautiful sight.
Of all that God has created for me.
The flowers, the mountains, and birds to hear and see.
I want to enjoy my family and friends
And not crawl in a hole as if the world ends.
To make new memories of those that are here.
And share your memory with those that care.
So I must make plans for the months to come.
Each morning greet with a happy welcome.
That I will take one day at a time.
And focus not on your death but the life of mine.
I will mourn my loss of you my son.
Forget how you died and all that was done.
It won't bring you back or erase my pain.
Your death broke my heart which now bears the stain.
I will miss you until the day I die.
Tears will be shed for you, I cry.
Until that day when my grief will end.
Then we will be together my son, my friend.

I Don't Understand If It Was God's Plan

I don't understand why you had to go.
I don't think that I will ever know.
I don't believe that it was part of God's plan.
For you to die by your own hand
I think God saw the pain you were in.
That you fought the battle and wouldn't win.
So he took your hand and helped you across.
Over to his side with others we lost.
Where you could no longer suffer in pain.
Where the sun always shines and there is no rain.
No struggles at work, no longer the fights.
No worries of finances and unpleasant nights.
That is what I do hope was part of God's plan.
With others in heaven, my handsome young man.
Jesus died on the cross to forgive us our sins.
That was before we were born, long before our kins.
How would he know what sins to forgive us for?
Because he knew we would make mistakes even more.
He knew we would slip and fall along the way.
For he is always watching over us every day.
He gave us life so precious he didn't want us to take away.
But he held out love for those that felt
they couldn't live another day.
For they were sick and helpless and knew not what to do.
They didn't have the strength to fight it like you.
I have to believe that God was there and him safely home.
That he is at peace in heaven as an angel, may he roam.

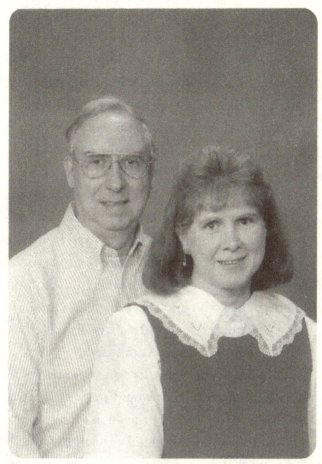
Michael's parents

Unanswered Questions Haunt Us Now

Unanswered questions haunt us now.
Asking why, and knowing how.
What happened to our child that day?
To make them feel they had to die that way,
To end their life and break our heart.
The pain so deep we fall apart.
Others tell us that we should move on.
Easy for them who still have their daughter or son.
They have no idea of the pain of walking in our shoes.
Until they lose a child they have no idea and have no clues.
There is no time table for our grief to end.
Better to offer their compassion and an ear to lend.
Than to tell us our child was selfish and unkind.
Or a coward, than one with a troubled mind.
Their pain was real and confused them so,
Their feelings were more like an enemy or foe.
If they had cancer, people would show more care,
But with suicide it's a secret they don't want to hear.
Maybe if they did, we wouldn't want to know,
About what they looked like or why they had to go.
Autopsies and police reports, do we really want to see.
Wondering if it will help eliminate the images haunting thee.
Why do we want to know those last details of their final days?
Knowing it could haunt us more in many painful ways.
Is this the way our life will be forever more?
Left with only memories of our child before?
Our patience gone, our smiles a frown.

Spend our day in a dressing gown.
No appetite, no desire to bathe or clean.
Grief rips our heart and leaves us mean.
Unanswered questions haunt us now.
Asking why and knowing how.
Only time and prayers will help us heal.
And telling others about how we feel.
But missing our child will never end or go away.
But hopefully our grief will end for us some day.

Shattered Dreams and Broken Hearts

Now that you are gone, how do I start?
To heal from my shattered dreams and broken heart.
Of the life I'd hoped you would fulfill,
Working hard all day developing your skill.
Wanting a family to call your own,
Because the one nearby made you feel alone.
Pressures of life too much to endure.
The financial worries of being left poor.
Depression mounted, your drinking increased,
Until your life you ended and now you're deceased.
My heart is now broken and I am all alone.
All I have left is my cries and a silent moan.
Since my child chose from this life to depart.
Leaving me with shattered dreams and a broken heart.

Are You Really There?

I know I'm in denial that my son is no longer here.
Yet I can't help but wonder as I call out "Are you really there?"
I know that pain eludes me and that I miss you so
But reality isn't here for me to accept your death you know.
I sometimes hear your laughter as I listen to a race.
But then I look to find you, but couldn't find you any place.
I once saw you in the airport, broke into tears immediately.
The sight of someone so like you, was startling for me.
Once sitting in the airport, across from me you sat.
Mustache upon the face, an earring too,
complete with baseball hat.
I wanted so much to go over to you and ask for a hug or two.
But then Brittany reminded me that it really wasn't you.
Yet why do I feel that it's all a lie and
that you are forever in eternity.
I can't believe you killed yourself and that
you are in heaven in reality.
I did not see you on that night, the coroner declared you dead.
A self-inflicted gunshot wound, you directed toward your head.
How easily you slipped away from those you loved that night.
A feeling of hopelessness and an end to
one's relentless need to fight
I know I'm glad I didn't see you die in such a way.
But I wished I could have hugged you and had the chance to say,
How much I really loved you and that I wanted you here with me.
That now you were with the angels living peacefully with thee.

Yet the closure it would have given me is no longer now to be.
The denial that it leaves me is something I must see
I must accept you are with the Lord and you are no longer here.
I must end the senseless wonder of "Are you really there?"

What if You Chose Your Family Like You Chose Your Friends?

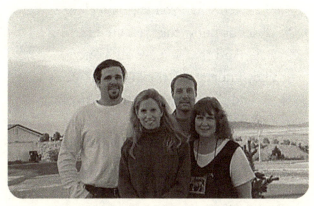

Michael with his stepbrother, Scott and stepsister, Lori and his mother, Linda

What if you chose your family
like you chose your friends?
Then maybe they would be there
When your heart needed to mend.
Families tend to squabble
And play head games with your heart.
Not caring if it hurts you
Or tears the family apart.
Friends take the time to call you
And inquire on how you are.
Where families will ignore you
Even though they don't live far.
True friends won't gang up on you
And leave you feeling blue.

They're always there to listen
Even when you leave no clue.
Friends know that you are grieving
And that you are all alone.
They understand the loss you suffered
And the pain that is full blown.
True friends are never jealous
Of the life that you have chose.
Not so with family who is always
Stepping on your toes.
If family would just treat you
Like your friends you treasure dear.
And be a comfort to you
And show they are sincere.
Just think how nice it would be,
If we chose our family like our friends.
To love one another sincerely
Like the Lord above recommends.

I try to think of all the pain that overwhelmed your day…

I try to think of all the pain
That overwhelmed your day.
That made you think that suicide
Would take it all away.
What was it on that day
That made you feel so blue?
It left you feeling hopeless
And feeling like dog-doo.
I think of how lonely and
How sad you must have been.
You had to be feeling all alone
Like in a lion's den.
Did you really know
What you were about to do?
Shooting yourself knowing
It would be the end of you.
Some say you were a coward
To do what you did.
But they didn't know the pain
Or the depression you hid.
I think it took a lot of courage
To end your life that way.
I can't believe that you planned to die
So close to Christmas day.
I wish I could turn back the clock
For you to have another chance.
To get the help and live your life,
And not give suicide a glance.

The Pain of Losing You

It's been seven months and eleven days
Without you here four major holidays.
The pain of losing you, and not having you here.
Left my heart broken and full of despair.
Asking all the questions, trying to make sense.
Putting on a false smile, living in pretense.
Going through the motions not know what to do.
Trying to understand why I'm left here mourning you.
I wake up in the morning no smile on my face.
Thoughts of you surround me unable to erase.
Visions of you embrace me, flooding my eyes.
Opening up the floodgates of tears from my cries.
Wishing you could be here to give me a hug.
Pulling your pranks on me, and feeling so smug.
How does a parent with their loss mend a broken heart?
When a child is taken from them their life is torn apart.
No one could ever take their place or fill the void it will leave.
No one can know the pain they're in for the child that they grieve.
Stop telling me that life goes on and that I must move on.
You didn't lose a child; it's my child that is gone.
You don't know the heartache or feel any of pain.
I shouldn't have to hear it or have to explain.
You only need to listen and let me know you're there.
When things get overwhelming and I need to know you care.
I know in time my heart will heal and I may smile for you.
And that my heart won't always feel like it is broken in two

What If's?

What if you didn't die and make your mother cry?
Didn't you know you would break my
heart when you chose to die?
What if you hadn't married or chose a different wife?
Would it have really mattered or even changed your life?
What if you had fathered your own children to raise?
Could you have handled the conflicts and given them praise?
Were you unable to handle the pressures and stress?
Overwhelming problems and depression too much to possess.
What if I lived closer so we could have gotten together?
Vacations at the beach in any kind of weather.
Would my move have mattered for you or made things right?
Or would your problems continue and end up in a fight?
So many questions left unanswered now by you.
Wondering what if any there was for us to do.
To get you the help you needed to keep you here with us.
Instead of feeling lonely and so helpless, unable to discuss.
Leaving those you left behind to ask all the What If's?

Grief...

Grief hits you like a bullet,
Shot deep into your heart.
It leaves you feeling breathless
And your heart torn all apart.
It feels like you're ripped open,
Exposed for all to see.
When all you want to do is crawl into a hole,
Where no one else can be.
No one can understand your grief,
Or understand the pain you're in.
Though they may say they do,
Their ignorance pricks you like a pin.
Grief leaves you feeling lonely
And some don't know what to do.
When all they really need to do,
Is to patiently listen to you.
Grief has no given number
Of how long some one should grieve.
The loss of your child
Too much for others to conceive.
The way they died causing pain,
For words once used before.
Giving it new meaning,
That now we must ignore.
Grief hits you like a bullet,
Shot deep into your heart.
It leaves you feeling breathless
And your heart torn all apart.

The Myth of Suicide
Thinking It Was a Sin

Why focus on the way one dies as if suicide was a sin.
Instead think of it as an illness that they were suffering in.
No need for shame for those who chose to self- inflict their end.
Instead reach out a hand to those they left, a parent or a friend.
Listen to them shed their tears and share their story with you.
Sometimes the only thing they need is someone to listen to.
The pain of losing someone so precious and dear to thee,
One only needs to know that others care and love you patiently.
It doesn't really help them to hear you understand how they feel.
You have no way of really knowing until it
has happened to you and it's real.
Don't tell them that their child was wrong or that they are in hell.
No one has ever returned from heaven or
hell, so how can you really tell.
I know my God is a loving God and that he loved us all.
He didn't cause my child's death; in his grace he didn't fall.
My God was a forgiving God who loved the sick and poor.
The truth is he really cared for them and loved them even more.
He gave them love and wanted them to reach out in a prayer.
And ask for help for those He gave to shower us with prayer.
The answer as to why they died is not for us to know.
Until our time is up on earth and heaven is where we go.
The myth of suicide in long years past
thought that it was a horrible sin.

Religion input their interpretations, which since
has been corrected, to fit the times we're in.
To understand the emotions and the sickness
that many suffered so quietly.
Undiagnosed and left untreated, the signs
were missed unfortunately.
We need to treat those contemplating
suicide with compassion tenderly.
Because one wouldn't shun the patient
who dies of cancer painfully.
Cause in the end the one who died left family here in pain.
They don't deserve to be left alone uncomforted in the rain.
Because their child chose to end their life
and hopelessness they're in.
Doesn't mean that those they left behind
need to be told it was a sin.

Healing Leaving Me With Out Feeling....

How long does it take for my grief to be healing?
Why do I linger in numbness without any feeling?
Unable to think of my son being dead,
Yet knowing he shot himself in his head.
Keeping myself busy to block out the pain.
May only delay my grieving, causing me no gain.
Doctor's say my pain is too much and my body isn't ready.
Nature's way of giving me time until my body isn't unsteady.
Amazing how it knows the devastation this loss will be.
Losing my only child, who was so precious to me.
I know in my heart, there is nothing I can do.
I can't go back in time and fix things for me or you.
I know I must face each day as a blessing from above.
I know I must be there for those that are here that I love.
I try to help others and share what I know.
Understanding suicide; recognizing the signs others may show.
If only to save one parent the pain a suicide leaves behind
Hurting inside because I didn't know this to save my son, so kind.
By joining a support group, we're sharing our story.
Of our children whose life ended without any glory.
We pour out our hearts and comfort each other.
In ways that we wished we could do with our mother.
But many of us have found that our family isn't there.
They give us no comfort and act like they don't care.
No mention of our children's name as if they were never here.
But their death to us was shattering because they were so dear.

How little do they realize how much we need to hear?
How much they miss our child and that they wish they were here.
Why is it so hard for people to express their feelings or fears?
Avoiding us just hurts us more as if no one really cares.
Yet here I sit and wonder if this grieving ever ends.
The pain of suicide horrific to the families, reeling in the winds.
Not wanting to forget them, a part of us gone.
Time shared on earth with them was not very long.
Why wouldn't we feel numb and left with no feeling?
Our life turned upside with our heart cold and reeling.
Living each day without any emotions.
The numbness of "going through the motions."
Like clouds drifting in the wind above.
Reminding us of the child we lost and we loved.
Our life is a circle that we are part of.
All part of a mystery from someone above.
I pray that his love will surround me each day.
Helping my grieving for my child to go away.
Leaving me with happier memories of a child dear to me.
Broken hearted by the world, yet no one could see.

Depression Is An Illness

Depression is an illness suffered by many these days.
Treatment is there for them in various ways.
Medication is used to treat their highs and lows.
Counseling therapies are held for many that goes.
Sometimes they get better and live normal lives.
With those that they care about, helping them thrive.
But then there are those that sink lower in despair.
Not reaching out to ones in their lives that care.
Left unattended and burdened with pain.
Denying the help their condition remains.
Where no one knows how to help them or knows of the signs.
Because mental illness means something is wrong with the mind.
The stigma it brings makes one want to hide.
Their symptoms increased left untreated inside.
We need more compassion and understanding these days.
The struggles of mankind continue in so many ways.
The pressure one's under no one has determined.
How much one can handle has not been examined.
If we knew what to look for we may be helpful to them.
Maybe encourage them treatment and be of comfort to them.
The hope that we give them to not face it alone.
That all of their friends are as close as a phone.
Instead of feeling alone with no future in sight.
They need to know that their suicide would never be right.
If only they waited for just one more day.
They would realize we loved them and help show them a way.
So learn what to look for and then you will know.
In case someone you love feels that they have to go.
Where life isn't a struggle and they will be at peace.
From the pain that their death will bring them release.

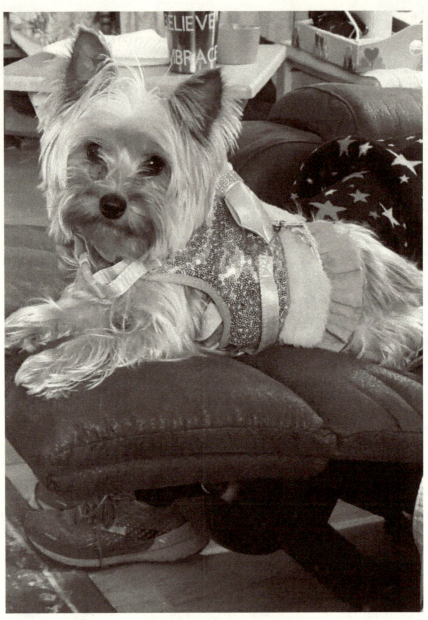

Caiterina Marie, Yorkshire Terrier, born Sept.22, 2021 has won my heart and helps with my depression and PTSD

Release Me From My Grief

Release me from the grief I'm in.
A new life for me I must begin.
The memory of my child that died.
Will always be with me and never set aside.
The lessons I've learned from his death will be
Helping others to learn what was unknown to me.
To help bring awareness to others in need.
That prevention of suicide is needed indeed.
To help spread the word around the world to all.
Depression leads to suicide, an illness, they fall.
Too many are suffering and dying at their own hand.
Their depression kept hidden feeling they wore a brand.
We must end this stigma and give them our love.
That help is available and God cares from above.
That there is a better solution if one only reaches out.
We all need to listen and all give a shout.
We all live in One Nation, Under God,
with Liberty, Justice for All.
To ignore suicide as an illness, is not anyone's call.
So I thank the Lord for all the help he has given me.
Release me from my grief, allowing me
to help others educationally.

My Son, He Was No Angel....
Till Now

My son, he was no angel, of this I do know.
Despite all his short-comings, his love he always did show.
He always acted impulsively, mistakes he did make.
Not thinking of the consequences, the risks he did take.
He accepted the outcome, no complaints did he voice.
Never blaming others for his actions, he knew was his choice.
If only he was able to control the impulsive act.
To think of the consequences in time to react.
His life would have been easier, no need for distress.
The peace that he needed, from all of the stress.
The depression he felt was more than we knew.
Bipolar disorder left untreated, his depression grew.
I knew nothing about it, the disorder unknown.
But the signs of the ups and downs, I now see were shown.
Resulting in his death, because he could see no other way.
To end all his suffering and unhappiness that dreadful day.
His feelings of failure, disappointment with life.
Alcohol count quite high, tired of the screams from his wife.
Though he was seen as strong, a muscular built man.
We failed to see how sensitive and insecure he felt as a man.
Told that men mustn't cry as they have to be strong.
When we know that hiding emotions is definitely wrong.
Hind-sight is no comfort to me now that he's gone.
Now living without my husband or son, I'm living alone.
My son was no angel on earth, this I know.
But now he is in heaven, an angel watching over me below.

Love Lost, Love Taken Away

Two lives held together by love so divine.
Soul mates together with their love would define.
What happened to end all the love that they had.
In such a short time, when did their love turn to bad?
Struggling to do well was all that he did.
The pain of his marriage failing he hid.
The family he loved so deeply failed him so
Feeling alone and forsaken, his beloved dared him to go.
Harsh words that were spoken from ones that once loved.
He turned to the bottle, felt betrayed by his beloved.
The fighting and screaming left him feeling trapped in a cage.
Feeling rejected, his life he had taken one night in a rage.
Love Lost…Love Hurts…Love Gone…Love Taken Away
Love Lost…Love Hurts…Love Gone…Life Taken Away
How can you love someone and call him your soul?
Yet treat him so poorly that he feels so much woe.
Knowing he was hurting, depressed every day.
No wonder he felt that death was his only way.
Harsh words they were spoken, the love it did lack.
Raised to not hit a woman, he didn't hit back.
The pain of his heartbreak expressed in his call.
He felt so alone and rejected by all.
Made to feel so unwanted with having no say.
Unable to discipline the kids, they went their own way.
Working hard to provide for them was all that they cared.
Ignoring his depression, their love wasn't shared.
Love Lost…Love Hurts…Love Gone… Love Taken Away
Love Lost…Love Hurts…Love Gone… Life Taken Away

The song that they cherished was known as Soul Shine.
Was used in their marriage when they pledged to be thine.
What should have lasted a lifetime was ended in two.
Two hearts sworn together when they said "I Love You!"
The love that one swore to each other that day.
Should have continued to blossom in every way.
Treating each other respectfully, showing that you did care.
If you had, maybe then today my son would be here.
Two years in a marriage for a love held so dear.
Made to feel so unwanted, he didn't want to be here.
Three words spoke in anger that night, "I Dare You!"
He ended his life tragically, forever it's true.
Love Lost… Love Hurts…Love Gone…Love Taken Away
Love Lost…Love Hurts…Love Gone…Life Taken Away
Lives thrown in turmoil, the love tossed aside.
The words once were stated, true love will abide.
Now lost forever, those words cannot be taken away.
Because he now is at peace with God, in whom we all pray.
I am now left to wonder if only I had known.
I was left out of his problems, because he was grown.
No one felt it necessary to tell me of the trouble he was in.
Perhaps if they had, together we could have helped him.
Depressions a killer left unattended or ignored for too long.
Ignoring the signs, not taking them seriously is wrong.
Help is needed by loved ones to encourage medical care.
Learning more about depression is needed everywhere.

A Year Without You Now

December 20 will be a year without you
Still hard to accept that your death is true
The shock of it all is too hard to accept.
The pain of the loss is felt to the depths.
Sometimes I feel so numb as if in a daze.
Unable to feel emotions, I stare in empty gaze.
Then there are days that tears fall in streams.
Nightmares replacing what used to be dreams.
Wake up mornings to the beautiful sunlight.
In spite of my efforts, no desire in sight.
To do what one used to find joy in before.
One's zest for life is no longer felt anymore.
I go through the motions of living as if I'm alive.
With none of the joy that once used to thrive.
I must accept that my son is now at peace.
His struggles and his depression now cease.
He didn't intend me to suffer from his choice.
He wanted me to live life full and rejoice.
But it isn't as easy as one might think.
My life without my son really does stink.
In time may it lesson and allow me to live on.
Life with some meaning, here without my son.
I need to keep busy and not dwell on my loss now.
To give my life some purpose without him somehow.

My Daughter, How Tragic Your Death Was For Me

Dedicated to all parents on POS losing a daughter.

My daughter, how tragic your death was for me.
I'm sorry I missed your signs, why didn't I see?
How sad that you felt so helpless and blue.
Your pain overwhelming that so consumed you.
How alone you did feel on that tragic day.
Left feeling so hopeless, with nothing to say.
I do wish you had reached out to me.
I could have hugged you so dearly, my daughter, you see.
I miss you so badly, my heart it does ache.
So deeply it feels like it surely will break.
My dreams for your future have drifted away.
It seems so unreal that it feels like a nightmare or play.
That you've gone on a trip and will return on some day.
Though I know you have died, I want you
back here with me, forever to stay.
My beautiful daughter so precious to me.
Now broken and lost to what life used to be.
How sadly I feel that you are no longer here.
I won't get to see you until I die and I'm there.
With you and the Lord, may you now be at peace.
May his love now surround you, your loneliness cease.
I treasure my memories of my life once with you.
Before your life turned upside down, and left you broken in two.
My beautiful daughter, I miss your smile and
laughter, and I'll always love you.

Life Is But A Passing....

In memory of my loving husband William D. Stilson
March 17, 1941 to February 2, 2001

Life is but a passing, of time upon this earth,
Time spent with one's beloved, sitting by the hearth,
Of holding hands together, while walking on the beach,
Knowing not how long one had, our fate was out of reach.
We spent our time together; complete our love did grow.
We thought we'd live forever, but little did we know.
My beloved was struck with cancer, and told that he would die,
Leaving me alone to mourn him and never asking why!
Instead I thank the good Lord, for all the time we had,
Cause in the end his illness had left him really bad.
We had the time to reminisce and say our "I Love You",
To use the time so precious, to pledge our love so true.
I use the strength he gave me to make it through each day,
To live my life its' fullest and take the time to pray.
Thank God for all the friends and family left behind for me,
And most of all I thank him for my memories with thee.

Published by Noble House Publishers London
2003 in "Theatre of the Mind"

I lost my husband to cancer Feb. 2, 2001. We had almost 27 years of marriage. We were at the prime of our life having just retired two years before he came down sick. I am proud of the way my husband handled his illness without complaining or feeling sorry for himself. He faced it head-on with strength and courage. That is why I take each day one day at a time and let others know I love them today. Don't put off until tomorrow because you don't know if you have a tomorrow. Knowing he was going to die, it gave us the time to say all that we wanted each other to know and not leave any loose ends. He was my love and my best friend. Before he died, we bought ATVs so that we had one last hobby to share and make lasting pleasant memories of his remaining six months. My son was terribly depressed, he knew how much I loved him and he told me how much he loved me and appreciated my always loving him despite his mistakes and for being there to help him out. I just wasn't able to help him out in the end, as he wasn't able to reach out to me when he was at his deepest sorrow. His death was devastating to me. One never knows when their time is up. So live life, laugh, and love.

Prayers Unending

Do you worry about our world,
Where angry words at others are hurled?
Where innocent are left to cry,
As others ask the question, why?

Have we come so far to only stray,
From our beliefs and prayer each day?
Why must it take a tragedy ending,
For us to give our prayers unending?

It's then we show our pride and solidarity,,
As we struggle to bring hope and prosperity.
Our being kind and thoughtful of each other,
By showing respect to one another.

Written by Linda J. Stilson after Sept. 11, 2001 attack on NYC
Copyright ©2003
Published in "The Layers Of Our Lives" in
USA By International Library of Poetry

I Had A Friend

In memory of Jeanine DuCharme
June 28, 1952 -July 15, 2002

I had a friend, so dear to me
That now I'll never see.
But I'll keep her memory close at heart
As though we weren't apart.
I'll think of her with laughter
Of the times I spent with her.
The smile she had would light the sky
Where now her soul will fly.
I know not why she had to go
As only God will know.
He saw her suffering and her pain
And brought her home, until we meet again.
For now she is at peace with him
An Angel now, rejoices in hymn.
For this is a painful journey we're on.
A tragic loss that one hadn't counted upon.
We cling to the faith of His Master Plan.
To be with him in Heaven with woman and man.
One step closer to those gone before.
Life without sorrow or tears anymore.

Jeanine was my best friend and she was depressed over having to move again and didn't want to move out of AZ. She was overwhelmed by many things that were going on in her life at that time. She sank deeper into depression and died of a heart attack. I think her heart was broken. She left behind a young daughter and son and a husband.

Grandma's Are Special And Fun To Be With

Dedicated to my Grandma Edna Hilligus and Grandma Eva Rounsville

A Grandma is special and fun to be with.
One that you love to visit or where you could live.
She teaches you to cook good things to eat.
You measure the ingredients and get to beat.
A Grandma has time for playing games.
Loves to call you silly names.
You get to dance and sing and play.
Lots of fun new things to do each day.
When I grow up I hope to be.
The way my Grandma was to me.
That is the legacy a Grandma leaves.
Leaving us memories of all that she believes.
May you be blessed with a Grandma like mine.
The greatest lady, so gracious and fine.
She makes me feel so special and warms my heart.
I know I will miss her, when we are apart.
My Grandma is special, sweet, and smart.

My Little Blessings

My granddaughter, Ashley has two sons, Noah Michael and Owen James who live nearby. She is a great help for me. I am blessed to have my great-grandsons come over to spend the day or have a sleepover. They give me something to look forward to and they help with my depression and living alone, just as my grandchildren did when I lost my husband and son. The boys have a lot of fun together playing games, creating art, using Ipads, playing outdoors and many more fun activites. I have a great-granddaughter in Hawaii that I hope to get to visit in a couple years.

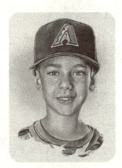

Noah Michael Morgan

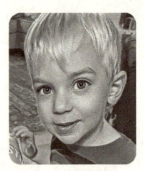

Owen James Morgan

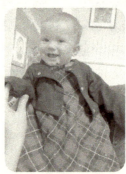

Lucille Lynn Quintana

Grief

GRIEF vs MOURNING

GRIEF is the internal experience of loss; the thoughts and feelings about a loss that you experience within yourself.

MOURNING is the outward expression of grief. Crying, talking about the person who died, or celebrating memories and anniversary dates are all ways of mourning.

"At times, we must grieve alone, but mourning is also necessary so that you are not alone."

The above information was obtained from http://www.uc.edu/psc/sh/SH_Grief.htm

MY GRIEF PROCESS:

Not everyone will experience all of these.

…Shock, denial, numbness, disbelief

This is where I am at. The reality of accepting my loss of my son is too painful for me and my body has put up what one calls "psychological shock absorbers" to protect me until I am ready to believe and handle my son's death. There is no time limit on this.

...Disorganization, confusion, searching, yearning:

My memory has suffered. I forget things and depend on a calendar or notepad. I went out to get the mail and came in the house only to go back out to check mail five minutes later. I once put the phone in the refrigerator, instead of on the base unit. I saw someone at the airport as I was getting ready to fly back for my son's service which caused me to breakdown. While waiting in Philadelphia airport with my twin granddaughters six months later, there was a guy sitting across from me that looked and dressed just like my son with a baseball hat on and looked just like him. My granddaughter pointed him out to me and asked if I was alright. I wanted to go over and hug the guy but then realized the guy might think I was crazy. These are referred to as "visual" hallucinations" and are considered normal responses to grief as well as dreams.

...Anxiety, panic, fear:

I started suffering anxiety attacks after my son died. I broke down in tears unexpectedly in front of a bank teller, who was very supportive. I broke down in Dillard's at the counter and was so emotional that I couldn't even talk. I had to write down for her to page my friend. One day I was at the dentist under nitrous oxide "laughing gas" and I broke down in tears so bad I couldn't breathe and started choking. I felt so bad for the dentist as I sure made it hard for him to work on my crown, but he was sympathetic.

This was all new for me during this grief as I didn't experience anxiety attacks when my husband died. I think it is because I took care of my husband at home and watched him suffer so it was a blessing, a relief, when he died.

…Physiological changes: loss of sleep, eating properly, self care

For two months after my son's death, I had trouble sleeping and was awakened at 3:15am. It then came to me that was the time my son was born.

My granddaughter, Brittany, called me at midnight one night worried about me eating. I had to make daily food reports to her for a couple weeks to tell her what I had to eat to alleviate her worries. I stayed in my nightgown most days as I had no desire to get dressed, unless I was going to church or with friends.

…Anger, resentment, jealousy, blame, terror, explosive emotions:

I have gone through the anger which sometimes leads to blame, but I know that neither will bring him back. I guess the resentment and jealousy for me was knowing that I won't have any "biological" grandchildren from him and that he was a part of me and there is no other part of him left for me now. I resented not being told more about my son's condition. I was his mother and deserved to know he was in trouble emotionally, but I know that they didn't know the signs anymore than I did. I blamed myself for not going back and demanding he get help, for not knowing the signs, and for not teaching him coping skills, if that was possible. It is so easy to go through the "what if's?" and to blame others or be angry with others or your child, however, none of it will bring back my son and so it isn't healthy for me to go that route, doesn't mean you don't have those feelings or that you don't experience them. I just don't dwell on them.

My twin granddaughter, Ashley, is mad at Michael for doing what he did knowing it has hurt me so. Children grieve just as adults and most often keep it to themselves. It is good to talk about it with them.

…Guilt:

As for guilt, I raised my son to know right from wrong and raised him as a Catholic. He went to church to complete his requirements and was Baptized, received his First Communion and was Confirmed. He wasn't raised to drink or break the law. I was a good mother and gave him my love as well as restrictions and consequences for his actions. He used to say he was "grounded for life". I did my best to raise him well. What I have had to accept is that he had choices to make and some choices have consequences. They were his choices, not mine. Guilt is divided up as:

…Survivor guilt -

I feel guilty that I didn't die instead. The death of my husband caused a rare liver disease I was born with to come out of remission which almost killed me twice. Why wasn't it my time? My son was only 33, why was it his time?

…Relief guilt -

I felt relief when my husband died because he had cancer and was in pain and I watched him suffer. I prayed that God would ease his pain.

My grief for my husband was different, losing my son was tragic.

The only relief that I can see for losing my son is that I don't have to worry about him struggling with life but that doesn't really provide me with any comfort or relief as I would rather he was here.

…Joy guilt -

I have found it difficult to feel happy after losing Michael.

However, I have grandchildren to make more memories with and lots of friends and family to spend time with. I have my church committees I am involved with as well as charity involvement within the community, and my Red Hat chapter ladies and friends to keep me busy. Sometimes keeping busy is helpful as long as it doesn't slow down your healing.

It is hard to feel joy at things I used to before, even though I know he wouldn't want me to be sad. His death wasn't about hurting me.

…Remorse and Regret:

I regret that I didn't know more about Bipolar Disorder in order to help my son. Yet I know that it would have been his choice to accept treatment and get help. I regret that my son was going through such a horrible time with me so far. I regret that my son isn't here to do the things that we talked about doing or the time that I wanted to have with him. I regret that I didn't go back to see for myself that he was doing better.

MY ADVISE ON HELPING PEOPLE WHO ARE GRIEVING THE LOSS OF A CHILD:

…Be there for support for them. Don't avoid them. Call them. Ask how they are doing. Invite them for lunch. Encourage them to get out, even if it is just for a ride in the car or a walk in the park. Ask if they need to talk.

…Don't give positive reasons from their loss. (Ex. No more worrying.)

…Don't suggest ways that the death could/should have been prevented. (Ex., If only.) It only implies blame.

…Don't make comparisons to the grief the survivor is experiencing to that of someone else you know or yourself. Their grief is about them, not you or someone else. They have just something very precious to them and it isn't the time to talk about yours or someone else's problems, or to make comparisons. Don't tell them how to grieve. Everyone grieves differently.

…Don't dwell on your own grief to show your sorrow. (Ex. Did you know that I tried to commit suicide? Or express that you are grieving more for the person than the survivor. This isn't about you, it is about their grief.

…Don't say that you know or understand what a parent is going through over the loss of their child. Only a parent who has lost a child can know their pain and understand. Everyone grieves differently, just as I did for my husband from grieving for my son.

…Expect that their will be emotional times and be prepared for them and listen. One doesn't have to talk. Just ask if you can give a hug and listen.

…Be willing to listen to them, sometimes that is all one wants. Mention their child's name and talk about some happy memories that you have of their child. Share funny stories of their child that they may not even know about.

…Don't take rejection by the survivor as personal attack and take into account the emotions that they are going through. They are not themselves.

…Don't tell them that their child was mean and a coward for committing suicide. Their child was obviously suffering and was not thinking clearly.

…Don't tell them how to grieve. For ex. , Don't tell them not to blame others or not to be angry. This is a process that they must go through and work out.

…Don't expect them to be over their grief at a specific time. Everyone grieves differently and it is common for some to have recurring grief.

…Once a parent has lost a child to suicide they become very sensitive to phrases that one once used but now it has painful meanings to them. For example, if someone lost a child by hanging, it is upsetting to hear the phrase "hanging around." For someone who committed suicide by gunshot, it is upsetting to hear the phrase "shoot myself in the foot" or other similar phrases referring to the use of shooting oneself. It helps to be cautious of what you are saying, as it now has new meaning for those grieving. My granddaughter, Brittany, doesn't want to watch movies with Christmas in it because my son committed suicide Dec. 20. She is also sensitive to movies that has shooting or death scenes in it. So it helps to think ahead to avoid any problems.

…Be sensitive to the parent that is grieving. They are more sensitive to remarks made and more likely to react out of anger. It is not a time to air your past issues. Remember this isn't about you; it is about their loss and pain. It is not the time. Most importantly, let them know that you care about them and keep in touch.

These are my grief processes that I have experienced. Just because one may feel anger or blame for someone, doesn't make it true. It is a normal emotion one is going through during their grief process. The suggestions are my suggestions and one must use their own judgment on what will be helpful for them in helping someone else. Remember each parent grieves differently.

Art Is My Therapy

I attend Occupational Therapy at the VAMC in Prescott, AZ three days a week where I get to'meet other veterans and make friends while we work on various mediums of art. I manly work on creating leather purses, backpacks, stools as well as mixed media canvass art, quilts, afghans and various art. Each year we can enter three pieces of art in the Northern Arizona Veterans Creative Arts Festival. I have been fortunate to have won 1st Place Regional on four homemade quilts, a crocheted afghan, mixed media canvas "Papa's Tools" and other mixed media canvas, five leather purses with one winning 2nd Place National. I won 1st Place Regional and 1st Place National on a copper relief of the Last Supper and a trip to Jacksonville Mississippi for a week full of activities and award ceremony. Art helps me with my depression and **PTSD**. **ART** is **THERAPY!**

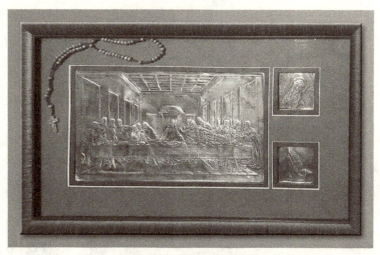

1st Place Regional and
National on copper relief of Last Supper

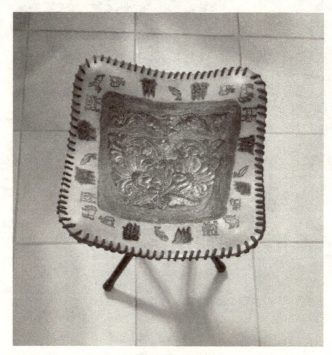

1st Place Regional
on leather stool for brother.

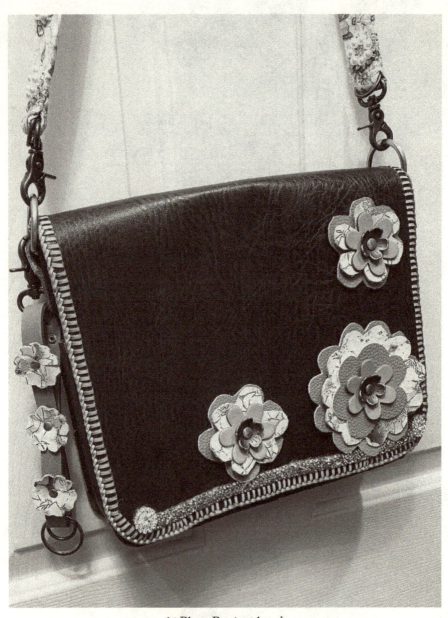

1st Place Regional and
2nd Place National on leather purse embellished with leather
Flowers with metal flower rivet in center of flower."

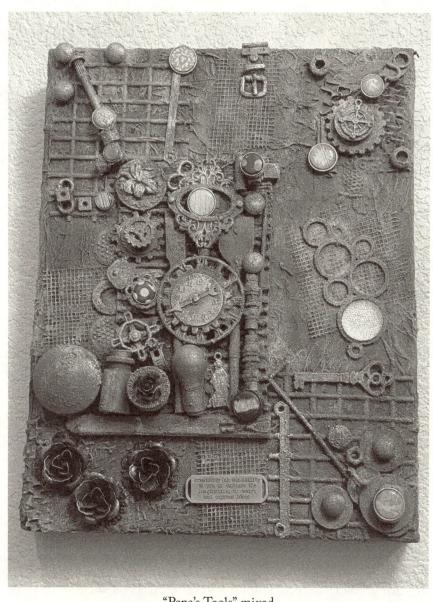

"Papa's Tools" mixed
Media canvass created with tools/parts found in my late
Husband's toolbox. Won 1st Place Regional.

American Association of SUICIDOLOGY

Dedicated To the Understanding
and Prevention of Suicide

WARNING SIGNS   Key Messages

Are you or someone you love at risk of suicide? Get the facts and take appropriate action. Get help immediately by contacting a mental health professional or calling 1-800-273-8255 for a referral should you witness, hear, or see anyone exhibiting any one or more of the following:

...Someone threatening to hurt or kill him/herself, or talking of wanting to hurt or kill him/herself.

...Someone looking for ways to kill him/herself by seeking access to firearms, available pills, or other means.

...Someone talking or writing about death, dying or suicide, when these actions are out of the ordinary for the person.

Seek help as soon as possible by contacting a mental health professional or calling 1-800-273-8255 for a referral should you witness, hear, or see someone you know exhibiting any one or more of the following:

...Hopelessness
...Rage, uncontrolled anger, seeking revenge

...Acting reckless or engaging in risky activities, seemingly without thinking
...Feeling trapped - like there's no way out
...Increasing alcohol or drug use
...Withdrawing from friends, family and society
...Anxiety, agitation, unable to sleep or sleeping all the time
...Dramatic mood changes
...No reason for living; no sense of purpose in life

American Association of Suicidology
5221 Wisconsin Avenue, NW
Washington, DC 20015
Phone: (202) 237-2280
Fax: (202) 237-2282
Email: info@suicidology.org
Website: www.suicidology.org

Facts about Suicide and Depression

FACTS ABOUT SUICIDE

In 2002, suicide was the eleventh leading cause of death in the U.S., claiming 31,655 lives. Suicide rates among youth (ages 15-24) have increased more than 200% in the last fifty years. The suicide rate is highest for the elderly (ages 65+) than for any other age group.

Four times ore men than women complete suicide, but three times more women than men attempt suicide.

Suicide occurs across all ethnic, economic, social and age boundaries.

Many suicides are preventable. Most suicidal people desperately want to live; they are just unable to see alternatives to their problems.

Most suicidal people give definite warning signals of their suicidal intentions, but those in close contact are often unaware of the significances of these warnings or unsure what to do about them.

Talking about suicide does not cause someone to become suicidal.

Surviving family members not only suffer the loss of a loved one to suicide, but are also themselves at higher risk for suicide and emotional problems.

WHAT IS DEPRESSION?

Major Depressive Disorder (MDD) is the most prevalent mental health disorder. In the U.S., the lifetime risk for MDD is 16.6% according to a recent study (Kessler et al., 2005). According to the National Institute of Mental Health (NIMH), 9.5-% or 18.8 million American adults suffer from a depressive illness in any given year.

Common symptoms of depression, reoccurring almost every day for a period of two weeks or more:
...Depressed mood (e.g. feeling sad or empty)
...Lack of interest in previously enjoyable activities
...Significant weight loss or gain, or decrease or increase in appetite
...Insomnia or hypersomnia
...Agitation, restlessness, irritability
...Fatigue or loss of energy
...Feelings of worthlessness, hopelessness, guilt
...Inability to think or concentrate, or indecisiveness
...Recurrent thoughts of death, recurrent suicidal ideation, suicide attempt or plan for completing suicide

June 10, 2005

A family history of depression (e.g., a parent) increases the chances (11-fold) that a child in that family will also have depression.

The treatment of depression is effective 60 to 80% of the time. However, according to the World Health Organization (WHO), less than 25% of individuals with depression receive adequate treatment.

Depression often is accompanied by co-morbid (Co-occurring) mental disorders (such as alcohol or substance abuse) and, if left untreated, can lead to higher rates of recurrent episodes and higher rates of suicide.

The Link Between Depression and Suicide

Suicide is the major life-threatening complication of depression.

Major Depressive Disorder (MDD) is the psychiatric diagnosis most commonly associated with completed suicide. Lifetime risk of suicide among patients with untreated MDD is nearly 20% (Gotlib & Hammen, 2002).

About 2/3 of people who complete suicide are depressed at the time of their deaths.

In a study conducted in Finland, of 71 individuals who completed suicide and who had Major Depressive Disorder, only 45% were receiving treatment at the time of death and only a third of these were taking antidepressants (Isometsa et al., 1994).

About 7 out of every 100 men and 1 out of every

100 women who have been diagnosed with depression at some time in their lifetime will go on to complete suicide.

The risk of suicide in people with Major Depressive Disorder is about 20 times that of the general population.

Individuals who have had multiple episodes of depression are at greater risk for suicide than those who have had one episode.

People who have a dependence on alcohol or drugs in addition to being depressed are at greatest risk for suicide.

Individuals who are depressed and exhibit the following symptoms are at particular risk for suicide.
...Hopelessness
...Rage, uncontrolled anger, seeking revenge
...Acting reckless or engaging in risky activities, seemingly without thinking
...Feeling trapped - like there's no way out
...Increasing alcohol or drug use
...Withdrawing from friends, family and society
...Anxiety, agitation, unable to sleep or sleeping all the time
...Dramatic mood changes
...Expressing no reason for living; no sense of purpose in life

Treatment

The most commonly used treatments for depression are:

...Pharmacology (i.e. antidepressants)

...Psychotherapy

...Electroconvulsive Therapy (ECT)

The best treatment for depression is the combination of antidepressants and psychotherapy. A meta-analysis of 16 studies (Pampalions et al., 2004) demonstrated the advantages of combined treatment versus pharmaceutical treatment alone. One hypothesis is that therapy increases adherence to the antidepressant treatment.

Treatments are effective 60 to 80% of the time. The Collaborative Depression Study indicates that after a first episode, 70% recovered within 5 years (National Institute of Mental Health).

ANTIDEPRESSANTS and SUICIDE RISK

In short-term studies, there has been some evidence that children and adolescents taking antidepressants exhibit a risk of increased suicidal ideation and/or suicide behaviors (suicidality). Given this, the concern is that antidepressants could potentially lead to completed suicide.

The U.S. Food and Drug Administration (FDA) analyzed 24 trials that included over 4400 patients and concluded that the risk of suicidality in children and adolescents who were prescribed antidepressants was 4% twice the placebo risk of 2% (www.fda.gov).

As with any new prescription in children and adolescents, careful monitoring of symptoms and side-effects should be observed by an adult. Any changes in symptomatology should be reported to the prescribing physician.

More research is required to determine if antidepressants are related to suicidality in children, adolescents and adults.

FDA "BLACK BOX" WARNINGS

The Food and Drug Administration (FDA) is now requiring manufacturers of antidepressants to add a "black box" warning label describing the potential risks of suicidality and the need for close monitoring of anyone prescribed this type of pharmacotherapy. Further info available on www.suicidology.org

BE AWARE OF FEELINGS, THOUGHTS, AND BEHAVIORS

Nearly everyone at some time in his or her life thinks about suicide. Most everyone decides to live because they come to realize that the crisis they are experiencing is temporary, but death is not. On the other hand, people in the midst of a crisis often perceive their dilemma as inescapable and feel an utter loss of control. Frequently, they:

…Can't stop the pain

If you experience any of these feelings, get help!

…Can't think clearly

If you know someone who exhibits these feelings,

…Can't make decisions offer help!

…Can't see any way out

…Can't sleep, eat, or work

…Can't get out of the depression

…Can't make the sadness go away

…Can't see the possibility of change

…Can't see themselves as worthwhile

…Can't get someone's attention

…Can't seem to get control

TALK TO SOMEONE - YOU ARE NOT ALONE. CONTACT:

...A community mental health agency private therapist ...A

...A school counselor or psychologist family physician ...A

...A suicide prevention/crisis religious/spiritual leader ...A intervention center

American Association of Suicidology

The goal of the American Association of Suicidology (AAS) is to understand and prevent suicide. AAS promotes research, public awareness programs, education, and training for professionals, survivors, and all interested persons. AAS serves as a national clearinghouse for information on suicide. AAS has many resources and publications, which are available to its membership and the general public. For membership information, please contact:

American Association of Suicidology 5221 Wisconsin Avenue, NW Washington, DC 20015

Phone: (202) 237-2280

Fax: (202) 237-2282

Email: info@suicidology.org

Website: www.suicidology.org

References:

Gotlib, I. H. Hammon, C. L. (Eds.). (2002) Handbook of depression. New York: Guilford Press

Isometsa, E, T., Aro, H. M., Henriksson, M. M., Heikkinen, M. E., & Lonnquist, J. K., (1994). Suicide in major depression in different settings. Journal of Clinical Psychiatry, 55(12), p.523-527 Kessler, E. C., Berglund, P. Denier, O., Jin, R., & Walters, E. E. (2005).

Lifetime prevalence and age-of-onset distributions of DSM-IV disorders in the National Comorbidity Survey Replication. Archives of General Psychiatry, 62, p. 593

Pampallona, S., Bollini, P., Tibaldi, G., Kupelnick, B., & Munizza, C. (2004).

Combined pharmacotherapy and psychological treatment for depression.

A systematic review. Archives of General Psychiatry. 61 (7), p. 714-719

WEBSITES:
National Institute of mental Health (http://www.nimh.nih.gov/)
U.S. Food & Drug Administration (http://www.fda.gov/)

Survivors of Suicide Fact Sheet

A survivor of suicide is a family member or friend of a person who died by suicide.

Some Facts…

Survivors of suicide represent "the largest mental health casualties related to suicide" (Edwin Shneidman, PhD., AAS Founding President).

There are currently almost 31,000 suicides annually in the USA. It is estimated that for every suicide there are at least 6 survivors. Some suicidologists believe this to be a very conservative estimate.

Based on this estimate, approximately 5 million American became survivors of suicide in the last 25 years.

About Suicidal Grief

The loss of a loved one by suicide is often shocking, painful and unexpected. The grief that comes can be intense, complex, and long term. Grief work is an extremely individual and unique process; each person will experience it in their own way and at their own pace.

Grief does not follow a linear path. Furthermore, grief doesn't always move in a forward direction.

There is no time frame for grief. Survivors should not expect that their lives will return to their prior state. Survivors aim to adjust to life without their loved one.

Common emotions experienced in grief are:
  Shock

Denial
Pain
Guilt
Anger
Shame
Despair
Disbelief
Hopelessness
Stress
Sadness
Numbness
Rejection
Loneliness
Abandonment
Confusion
Self-blame
Anxiety
Helplessness Depression

These feelings are normal reactions and the expression of them is a natural part of grieving. At first, and periodically during the following day/months of grieving, survivors may feel overwhelmed by their emotions. It is important to take things one day at a time. Crying is the expression of sadness; it is therefore a natural reaction after the loss of a loved one.

August 30, 2004

Survivors often struggle with the reasons why the suicide occurred and whether they could have done something to prevent the suicide or help their loved one. Feelings of guilt typically ensue if the survivor believes their loved one's suicide could have been prevented.

At times, especially if the loved ones had a mental disorder, the survivor may experience relief.

There is a stigma attached to suicide, partly due to the misunderstanding surrounding it. As such, family members and friends of the survivor my not know what to say or how and when to provide assistance. They may rely on the survivor's initiative to talk about the loved one or to ask for help.

Same or embarrassment might prevent the survivor from reaching out for help. Stigma, ignorance and uncertainty might prevent family and friends from giving the necessary support and understanding. Ongoing support remains important to maintain family and friendship relations during the grieving process.

Survivors sometimes find that others are blaming them for the suicide. Survivors may feel the need to deny what happened or hide their feelings. This will most likely exacerbate and complicate the grieving process.

When the time is right, survivors will begin to enjoy life again. Healing does occur.

Many survivors feel that the best help comes from attending a support group for survivors of suicide where they can openly share their own story and their feelings with fellow survivors without pressure or fear of judgment and shame. Support groups can be a helpful source of guidance and understanding as well as a support in the healing process.

Children as Survivors

It is a myth that children don't grieve. Children may experience the same range of feelings as do adults; the expression of that grief might be different as children have fewer tools for communicating their feelings.

Children are especially vulnerable to feelings of guilt and abandonment. It is important for them to know that the death was not their fault and that someone is there to take care of them.

Secrecy about the suicide in the hopes of protecting children may cause further complications. Explain the situation and answer children's questions honestly and with age- appropriate responses.

American Association of Suicidology

The American Association of Suicidology (AAS) offers a variety of resources and programs to survivors in an attempt to lessen the pain as they travel their special path of grief. These include:

…Survivors of Suicide Kit: an information kit consisting of fact sheets, a bibliography and sample literature.
…Survivors of Suicide: Coping with the Suicide of a Loved One booklet and A Handbook for Survivors of Suicide.
…Surviving Suicide, a quarterly newsletter for survivors and survivor support groups.
…"Healing After Suicide", an annual conference held every April, for and about survivors.
…Suicide Prevention and Survivors of Suicide Resource Catalog: a listing of books, pamphlets, etc. which can be ordered from AAS. Includes resources for children and those who care for them.
,,,Directory of Survivors of Suicide Support Groups - print version

available for purchase and an online version available at www.suicidology.org

...Guidelines for Survivors of Suicide Support Groups: a how-to booklet on starting a support group.

Additional Resources

...American Foundation for Suicide Prevention (AFSP) (www.afsp.org).

...Survivors of Suicide (www.survivorsofsuicide.com).

...The Link National Resource Center (www.thelink.org).

BE AWARE OF THE WARNING SIGNS

WARNING SIGNS:

Are you or someone you love at risk of suicide? Get the facts and take appropriate action. Get help immediately by contacting a mental health professional or calling 1-800-273-8255 for a referral should you witness, hear, or see anyone exhibiting any one or more of the following:

…Someone threatening to hurt or kill him/herself, or talking of wanting to hurt or kill him/herself.

…Someone looking for ways to kill him/herself by seeking access to firearms, available pills, or other means.

…Someone talking or writing about death, dying or suicide, when these actions are out of the ordinary for the person.

Seek help as soon as possible by contacting a mental health professional or calling 1-800-273- 8255 for a referral should you witness, hear, or see someone you know exhibiting any one or more of the following:

…Hopelessness
…Rage, uncontrolled anger, seeking revenge
…Acting reckless or engaging in risky activities, seemingly without thinking
…Feeling trapped - like there's no way out
…Increasing alcohol or drug use
…Withdrawing from friends, family and society
…Anxiety, agitation, unable to sleep or sleeping all the time
…Dramatic mood changes
…No reason for living; no sense of purpose in life

Understanding and Helping the Suicidal Individual

BE AWARE OF THE FACTS

1. SUICIDE IS PREVENTABLE. Most suicidal individuals desperately want to live; they are just unable to see alternatives to their problems.

2. Most suicidal individuals give definite warnings of their suicidal intentions, but others are either unaware of the significance of these warnings or do not know how to respond to them.

3. Talking about suicide does not cause someone to be suicidal.

4. Approximately 32,000 Americans kill themselves every year. The number of suicide attempts is much greater and often results in serious injury.

5. Suicide is the third leading cause of death among young people ages 15-24, and it is the eighth leading cause of death among all persons.

6. Youth (15-24) suicide rates increased more than 200% from the 1950's to the late 1970's. Following the late 1970's, the rates for youth suicide have remained stable.

7. The suicide rate is higher among the elderly (over 65) than any other age group.

8. Four times as many men kill themselves as compared to women, yet three times as many women attempt suicide as compared to men.

9. Suicide cuts across all age, economic, social, and ethnic boundaries.

10. Firearms are currently the most utilized method of suicide by essentially all groups (male, female, young, old, white, non-white).

11. Surviving family members not only suffer the trauma of losing a loved one to suicide, and may themselves be at higher risk for suicide and emotional problems.

WAYS TO BE HELPFUL TO SOMEONE WHO IS THREATENING SUICIDE

1. Be aware. Learn the warning signs.

2. Get involved. Become available. Show interest and support.

3. Ask if he/she is thinking about suicide.

4. Be direct. Talk openly and freely about suicide.

5. Be willing to listen. Allow for expression of feelings. Accept the feelings.

6. Be non-judgmental. Don't debate whether suicide is right or wrong, or feelings are good or bad. Don't lecture on the value of life.

7. Don't dare him/her to do it.

8. Don't give advice by making decisions for someone else to tell them to behave differently.

9. Don't ask "why". This encourages defensiveness.

10. Offer empathy, not sympathy.

11. Don't act shocked. This creates distance.

12.   Don't be sworn to secrecy. Seek support.

13. Offer hope that alternatives are available, do not offer glib reassurance, it only proves you don't understand.

14. Take action! Remove means! Get help from individuals or agencies specializing in crisis intervention and suicide prevention.

BE AWARE OF FEELINGS, THOUGHTS, AND BEHAVIORS

Nearly everyone at some time in his or her life thinks about suicide. Most everyone decides to live because they come to realize that the crisis is temporary, but death is not. On the other hand, people in the midst of a crisis often perceive their dilemma as inescapable and feel an utter loss of control. Frequently they;

…Can't stop the pain

…Can't think clearly

…Can't make decisions

…Can't see any way out

…Can't sleep, eat, or work

…Can't get out of the depression

…Can't make the sadness go away

…Can't see the possibility of change

...Can't see themselves as worthwhile

...Can't get someone's attention

...Can't seem to get control

TALK TO SOMEONE - YOU ARE NOT ALONE CONTACT:

...A community mental health agency

...A school counselor or psychologist

...A suicide prevention/crisis intervention center

...A private therapist

...A family physician

...A religious/spiritual lender

The goal of the American Association of Suicidology (AAS) is to understand and prevent suicide. AAS promotes research, public awareness programs, education, and training for professionals, survivors, and all interested persons. AAS serves as a national clearinghouse for information on suicide. AAS has many resources and publications, which are available to its membership and the general public. For membership information, please contact:

American Association of Suicidology

5221 Wisconsin Avenue, NW

Washington, DC 20015

Phone: (202) 237-2280

Fax: (202) 237-2282

Email: info@suicidology.org Website: www.suicidology.org

The information on suicide signs, warnings, facts, depression, etc. was provided, with permission, from The American Association of Suicidology (AAS). Please check out their website for further information. I want to thank Kristin E. Bergeron, Research Assistant, at the American Association of Suicidology for her assistance in gaining permission to use their information to promote suicide awareness.

SUICIDE AWARENESS & PREVENTION:
Know the Signs *

People usually attempt suicide to bock unbearable emotional pain, which is caused by a wide variety of problems. It is often a cry for help. A person attempting suicide is often so distressed that they are unable to see that they have other options: we can help prevent a tragedy by endeavoring to understand how they feel and helping them to look for better choices that they could make. Suicidal people often feel terribly isolated; because of their distress, they may not think of anyone they can turn to, furthering this isolation. In the vast majority of cases a suicide attempter would choose differently if they were not in great distress and were able to evaluate their options objectively. Most suicidal people give warning signs in the hope that they will be rescued, because they are intent on stopping their emotional pain, not on dying.

The majority of individuals who commit suicide do not have a diagnosable mental illness. They are people just like you and I who at a particular time are feeling isolated, desperately unhappy and alone. Suicidal thoughts and actions may be the result of life's stresses and losses that the individual feels they just can't cope with.

People can usually deal with isolated stressful or traumatic events and experiences reasonably well, but when there is an accumulation of such events over an extended period, our normal coping strategies can be pushed to the limit.

The stress or trauma generated by a given event will vary from person to person depending on their background and how they deal with that particular stressor. Some people are personally more or less vulnerable to particular stressful events, and some people may find certain events stressful which others would see as a positive experience. Furthermore, individuals deal with stress and trauma in different ways; the presence of Multiple risk factors do not necessarily imply that a person will become suicidal.

RISK FACTORS that may contribute to a person feeling suicidal include:

Significant changes in Relationships.
...Well-being of self or family member.
...Body image.
...Job, school, university, house, locality.
...Financial situation.
...World environment.

Significant losses:
...Death of a loved one.
...Loss of a valued relationship.
...Loss of self esteem or personal expectations.
...Loss of employment. Perceived abuse:
...Physical

...Emotional/Psychological.
...Sexual
...Social
...Neglect

Often suicidal people will give warning signs, consciously or unconsciously, indicating that they need help and often in the hope that they will be rescued. These usually occur in clusters, so often several warning signs will be apparent. The presence of one or more of these warning signs is not intended as a guarantee that the person is suicidal; the only way to know for sure is to ask them. In other cases, a suicidal person may not want to be rescued, and may avoid giving warning signs.

TYPICAL WARNING SIGNS often exhibited by people who are feeling suicidal:

...Withdrawing from friends and family.
...Depression, broadly speaking; not necessarily a diagnosable mental illness such as clinical depression, but indicated by signs such as:
...Loss of interest in usual activities.
...Showing signs of sadness, hopelessness, irritability.
...Changes in appetite, weight, behavior, level of activity or sleep patterns.
...Loss of energy.
...Making negative comments about self.
...Recurring suicidal thoughts or fantasies.
...Sudden change from extreme depression to being "at peace" (may indicate that they have decided to attempt suicide).
...Talking, Writing, or Hinting about suicide.
...Previous attempts.
...Feelings of hopelessness and helplessness.
...Purposefully putting personal affairs in order:

…Giving away possessions.
…Sudden intense interest in personal wills or life insurance.
…"Clearing the air" over personal incidents from the past.
This list is not definitive: some people may show no signs yet still feel suicidal, others may show many signs yet be coping OK; the only way to know for sure is to ask.

In conjunction with the risk factors listed above, this list is intended to help people identify others who may be in need of support.

* This information was provided for me by Parents of Suicide (POS) to promote suicide awareness.

The following information on Catholic views on suicide was obtained from http://www.scborromeo.org/ccc.htm
From: The Second Edition English Translation of the Catechism of the Catholic Church

Suicide: Definition: The willful taking of one's own life; a grievous sin against the fifth commandment. A human person is neither the author nor the supreme arbiter of his life, of which God is sovereign master.

2281 Suicide contradicts the natural inclination of the human being to preserve and perpetuate his life. It is gravely contrary to the just love of self. It likewise offends love of neighbor because it unjustly breaks the ties of solidarity with family, nation, and other human societies to which we continue to have obligations. Suicide is contrary to love for the living God.

#2282 If suicide is committed with the intention of setting an example, especially to the young, it also takes on the gravity of scandal. Voluntary co-operation in suicide is contrary to the moral law.

Grave psychological disturbances, anguish, or grave fear of hardship, suffering, or torture can diminish the responsibility of the one committing suicide

2283 We should not despair of the eternal salvation of persons who have taken their own lives. By ways known to him alone, God can provide the opportunity for salutary repentance. The Church prays for persons who have taken their own lives.

Websites for Additional Information:

I wish I had been aware of these websites in time to save my son, so I hope it helps you to understand suicide and learn the signs to watch out for. I think that as a parent we need to accept that our children can't always cope with problems in life the same as others and we should be educated as well as the children in school.before it is too late.

American Foundation of Suicide Prevention (888) 333-AFSP
http://www.afsp.org http://www.yellowribbon.org

American Association of Suicidology
1-800-273-8255
http://www.suicidology.org/survivorsofsuicide. htm
http://www.suicidology.org/index.cfm Dedicated to the understanding and prevention of suicide. Promotes research, public awareness programs, education and training. Web site has info on support groups.

Suicide Prevention Awareness Network (SPAN) http://www.spanusa.org

Survivors of Suicide http://www.survivorsofsuicide.com/
Provides lots of information on suicide as well as support groups. Directory of support groups. Poetry submitted by survivors.
11Death is not the greatest loss in life. The greatest loss is what dies inside us while we live.11

Depression http://www.depression.com

Bipolar Disorder http://www.bipolar.com

National Institute of Mental Health-info on depression and bipolar disorder http://www.nimh.nih.gov/publicat/bipolar.cfm

Department of Health and Human Services, Centers for Disease Control and Prevention.info on suicide

http://www.cdc.gov

Yellow Ribbon group which focuses on teen suicide prevention. http://www.yellowribbon.org

Suicide Support Prevention, Awareness Education, Survivors http://www.geocities.com/tlcprojects2001/proje ct43

Suicide and Self-Injury Resources http://www.depression.about.com/od/suicide

Suicide Awareness Voices of Education (SAVE) http://www.save.org/coping/
Suicide Reference Library www.suicidereferencelibrary.com

The Compassionate Friends http://www.compassionatefriends.org/ assist families toward the positive resolution of grief following the death of a child of any age and to provide information to help others be supportive.

ONLINE SUPPORT GROUPS :

Parents of Suicide (POS) online support group for parents who have lost a child to suicide
Email to subscribe: subscribe@yahoogroups.com http://www.parentsofsuicide.com

Friends & Families of Suicides (FFOS) online support group for friends and families who have lost a child to suicide www.friendsandfamiliesofsuicide.com

Grieving Siblings (GS) a group of young women ages 15-25 who have lost brothers or sisters.
Send email to: subscribe@yahoogroups.com

Suicide Awareness Education and Support (SASE)
Send email to: subscribe@yahoogroups.com Suicide Discussion Board, A place for Support and Healing after a suicide.is open for the purpose of suicide awareness, support and education for those whose lives have been affected by suicide. .Parents of Suicide (POS) and Suicide Awareness Education and Support (SASE) www.suicidediscussionboard.com/viewtopic.ph p

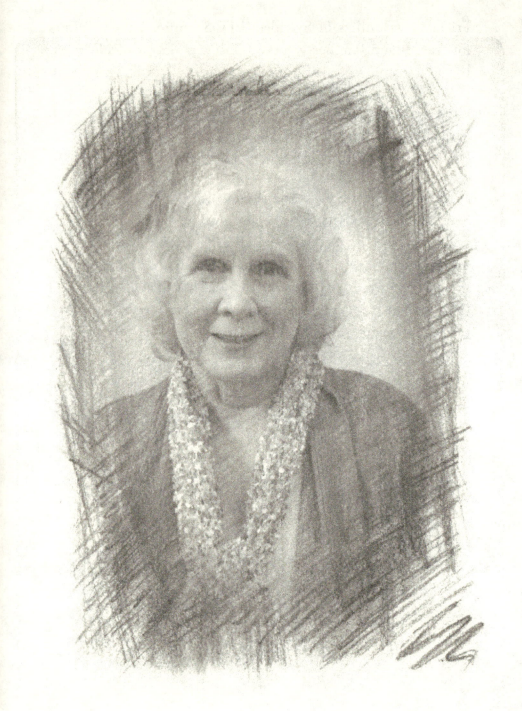

Printed in the USA
CPSIA information can be obtained
at www.ICGtesting.com
LVHW091638190924
791537LV00045B/351